HERBS FOR

The author of this book is a practising herbalist, naturopath and osteopath, and, as first woman President of the National Institute of Medical Herbalists, she has broadcast over national radio and TV on herbalism. Here she describes and explains how to use twenty-five different herbs in the treatment of colds and 'flu and their after effects.

HERBS
FOR
COLDS AND 'FLU

by
NALDA GOSLING
F.N.I.M.H., M.B.N.O.A., N.D., D.O.

Drawings by A.R. Gosling

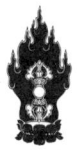

1981 SHAMBHALA *Boulder*

SHAMBHALA PUBLICATIONS, INC.
1920 Thirteenth Street
Boulder, Colorado 80302

© 1976 by Nalda Gosling
All rights reserved

Published by arrangement with Thorson Publishers, Ltd.
Distributed by Random House

Printed in the United States of America

Library of Congress Cataloging in Publication Data
Gosling, Nalda.
  Herbs for colds and 'flu.

  (Everybody's home herbal)
  Includes index.
  1. Cold (Disease) 2. Influenza. 3. Herbs—
Therapeutic use. I. Title.
RF361.G67   1981   616.2'03061   80-53450
ISBN 0-87773-203-5 (pbk.)
ISBN 0-394-74834-4 (Random House: pbk.)

CONTENTS

		Page
	Introduction	7
1.	Preventative Measures	10
2.	Remedial Treatment	19
3.	Agrimony	23
4.	Avens	25
5.	Balm	27
6.	Bayberry	28
7.	Boneset	30
8.	Catmint	31
9.	Cayenne	33
10.	Clivers	34
11.	Coltsfoot	36
12.	Echinacea	37
13.	Elder	39
14.	Garlic	41
15.	Golden Rod	43
16.	White Horehound	44
17.	Hyssop	45
18.	Lime Flowers	46
19.	Meadowsweet	48
20.	Oats	49
21.	Pleurisy Root	51
22.	Rosemary	52
23.	Sage	54
24.	Sweet Flag	56
25.	Tansy	58
26.	Vervain	59
27.	Yarrow	61
	Therapeutic Index	62

INTRODUCTION

Influenza and the common cold, although apparently simple conditions of usually limited duration, could almost be considered to be a plague on mankind.

It has been calculated that the common cold may cost Great Britain about £700 million per year, assessing an average of seven days' loss of work for each worker. Influenza, which may necessitate absence from work of anything between three days and five or six weeks, not only costs much more to the economy of the country but kills about 3,000 people each year; more when there is a serious epidemic!

It is an illness which presents particular hazards to the very young and the old, and may lead on to broncho-pneumonia or leave a legacy of weakened heart muscle.

The Common Cold

There must be few people who have never experienced a common cold, with the symptomatic dry, sore throat, a streaming nose, reddened eyes, loss of smell and taste, the feeling of being 'out of sorts', and probable subsequent naso-pharyngeal catarrh.

In spite of intensive research for almost thirty years, no definite conclusions on cause and cure of the common cold have been reached. The orthodox theory is that a germ or virus attacks the nasal mucosa – the lining of the nose – setting up a localized inflammatory state which may extend along the mucous membrane lining of the upper respiratory passages. This may lead to slightly raised temperature, and the inflammatory state may affect the bronchial passages, causing a cough and perhaps bronchitis.

Experiments carried out at the Common Cold Research Unit, in which attempts are made to transmit a cold by applying a live virus into the nostrils of volunteers, have not fully confirmed this theory, in that not all the persons developed a cold. It is still unknown to the researchers why some people will be susceptible to colds and others not.

Influenza

This infectious fever can be devastating in its effects, reaching epidemic or pandemic proportions. The most notable pandemic this century was that of 1918/19, when influenza swept across western Europe and Britain, its effects becoming world-wide. In all twenty million people died, either from the influenza itself or from its subsequent complications.

Research has indicated that the viral background of influenza is complex; the disease is due to virus of three types, A, B or C, each one of which is variable. Resistance may build up in the individual following an attack of influenza, but that resistance will apply only to the same strain of virus or a related strain, not to a different type. Epidemics of influenza usually develop in waves; type A, 'Asian' 'flu (the most virulent type), develops about every ten years, as witness the pandemic which originated in China in 1957 and the 'Hong Kong' 'flu of 1968.

Asian 'flu was a particularly hazardous type; about eighty million cases were reported. Virus A infects pigs, horses and birds as well as humans, and may cause outbreaks or epidemics every two or three years, perhaps affecting 10 per cent of the population in a milder infection than Asian-type influenza. Virus B is the most variable, but is usually less extreme than Asian virus type A. Virus C causes a milder type of influenza.

Vaccines

Orthodox treatment for colds and influenza consist of vaccines – which must exactly match the virus – or pain-killers, of which the most common are aspirin and paracetamol; decongestants which may be either adrenaline derivatives or antihistamines; drying agents such as belladonna; cough-suppressants which are derived from morphine-like drugs, or expectorants to disperse mucus from the bronchial tubes. None of these methods, when combined with the normal attitude towards diet, can be considered to provide success in creating a healthier nation.

Vaccine manufacturers need to play a guessing game as to which type of virus will appear next, and they find it is extremely difficult to produce sufficient vaccine of the correct strain when an epidemic has suddenly developed. A pain-killer such as aspirin brings its own hazards of irritating the gastric mucosa, and the cough-suppressant may lead to chronic bronchial diseases such as emphysema, due to the dried mucus residual in the bronchial tubes.

1.

PREVENTATIVE MEASURES

Far wiser than the wild search for viruses and their antagonists is the principle of prevention. By building up a good standard of health, resistance against infection is increased. The body has its own natural immunity which may be implemented by wise measures. There are many plants which are useful in aiding the building of good health.

The naturopath believes that colds, catarrh and allied conditions are an attempt by the body to rid itself of toxins and waste, usually the accumulation of a faulty diet which has been overwhelmed with carbohydrates, white sugar and white flour products, and an inadequate quantity of fresh fruit, salads and vegetables.

The digestive system becomes incapable of dealing with the starchy wastes, the tissues become clogged, there is often associated constipation due to inadequate roughage, and a 'cold' results. Many previous sufferers from frequent colds, recurrent or constant catarrh and a dripping nose, have experienced the benefit of a short fast on fruit juices, leading to a balanced diet of salads, fresh fruits, and vegetables raw or conservatively cooked, protein, wholewheat bread and a minimum of brown sugar or honey. General health and vitality improve, the constant colds and catarrh become merely a memory.

Two Natural Remedies

This type of diet may be supplemented with garlic (see page 41) and vitamin C. These may be taken during the winter only, when there is normally less resistance, or in severe cases, where hay-fever or bronchial conditions may be a complication, they can be introduced at any time of the year.

Garlic is not offensive when taken in capsule form; the oil is deodorized and is hardly noticed on the breath. Two or three capsules at bedtime should be adequate.

Vitamin C, or ascorbic acid, was first discovered in 1928. It is known to provide resistance against colds and infections, to support the cells concerned with formation of bone and the enamel and dentine of teeth, and is necessary for formation of intercellular connecting protein collagen, hence its value in rheumatism and allied conditions. The major disease associated with deficiency of this vitamin is scurvy, characterized by swollen spongy gums and haemorrhages under the skin.

Much research has been undertaken into the value, uses and daily intake of vitamin C, and much controversy has arisen over the amount needed for good health. The quantity given by the Department of Health and Social Security in 1969 was 30mg for the adult man or woman, which is the amount present in 100g ($3\frac{1}{2}$oz.) of boiled sprouts. This quantity is challenged by the findings of Dr

Linus Pauling, Professor of Chemistry at Stanford University, California, and winner of two Nobel prizes.

Following many years of study and research into the uses of vitamin C, Dr Pauling recommends a regular intake of at least 250mg daily for optimum health, and suggests taking 500mg tablets every hour or two at the first sign of a cold or infection. He has used this vitamin (in what are considered by many physicians to be massive doses) for over ten years without any harmful effects. Szent-Györgyi, the man who first isolated vitamin C, has said: 'One can take any amount of ascorbic acid without the least danger.'

Control of Diet

Dr Pauling believes that most colds can be prevented or largely ameliorated by control of diet, without the use of drugs. The dietary substance involved is vitamin C. He says:

> I am sure that an increased intake of ascorbic acid leads to improvement in general health and to increased resistance to infectious disease, including the common cold.

Vitamin C is present in green vegetables, fruits, tomatoes and potatoes, one of the finest sources being blackcurrant at 200mg per 100g. Oranges yield 50mg per 100g, and at the lower end of the scale pears give 2mg for every 100g. This vitamin is destroyed by exposure to air and heat, and up to 75 per cent of vitamin C in green vegetables may be lost in cooking.

Vegetables should be cooked quickly in a minimum of boiling water, and should be taken out while still slightly crisp. Shredding them finely, although it loses some of the vitamin content, speeds the cooking process. Vegetables completely immersed in water may lose up to 80 per cent of vitamin C. A good source of the vitamin, providing controlled dosage, is either syrup or capsules, which are readily obtainable from health food stores.

Lemon Juice

In addition to blackcurrant or rose-hip, in capsule or syrup form, a useful source of Vitamin C is the lemon. The fruit contains 50mg vitamin C per 100g, and its juice may be taken diluted with hot water and sweetened with a little honey. Use this frequently at the first sign of a cold or influenza, and as a cool refreshing drink after the temperature has returned to normal.

A pleasant source of vitamin C, and also a thirst-quenching drink, is the juice of one lemon and the juice of three oranges, diluted to taste with water in which a little honey has been dissolved.

The lemon has astringent and antiseptic properties and can be used, in cold water, as a gargle for a sore throat or as a preventative gargle after possible contact with infection; perhaps after being amongst a crowd, or after a journey in a crowded bus or train in winter.

A few drops of lemon juice may be added to cold water to tone and cleanse the nostrils in persistent nasal catarrh. This may be sprayed into the nostrils or sniffed gently into each nostril in turn, and allowed to run out immediately.

Also as a preventative measure the juice of

half a lemon in hot water, with honey to sweeten, may be taken on rising or at bedtime.

Fresh Air
In discussing preventative measures commonsense must not be forgotten. Obviously one should avoid being wet and chilled or having cold feet for a prolonged time, but the sufferer from frequent colds will often avoid becoming chilled by wrapping up warmly and remaining indoors in warm rooms as much as possible. Such practice may appear to help, but in fact may lower the resistance to colds and chills.

It has been found that a regular daily routine of a brisk walk in the fresh air and a morning cold friction rub will stimulate and improve the circulation. The cold friction rub, which need only take five minutes, can be carried out with a loofah or body-brush dipped repeatedly in cold water and used to quickly rub with circular motion each limb in turn and then the body; rubbing dry briskly afterwards with a towel. This should impart a delightful glowing feeling, and is a superb start to the day.

Maintaining Vitality
Valuable in building up resistance to colds and infection is the ability to maintain vitality. This can be done in two major ways: firstly, by the commonsense measures of avoiding unnecessary fatigue, i.e. by ensuring adequate sleep and by refraining from extreme overwork. A succession of late nights and a tendency to work beyond the limits of

normal activity will drain reserve energy. At the same time the habit of remaining indoors in winter in stuffy, ill-ventilated and perhaps smoke-filled rooms – thus reducing oxygen intake – puts too great a load of acids and impurities on the circulation, and the way is prepared for the development of colds and infections.

The second factor, to which reference has already been made, is that of diet. Food which is rich in the essential nutritional elements – proteins, fats, vitamins and minerals with a minimum of carbohydrates – gives the body enough sustenance to carry out its normal work.

The vital criteria regarding health, and the adequacy or otherwise of diet, is that weight remains fairly constant; that there is enough energy to carry out the normal routine of work and some to spare; that appetite is good and is satisfied; that there is a good daily evacuation from the bowels, and that sleep comes easily and is refreshing. If any of these conditions are variable without known cause the reason must be sought.

Obesity

Obesity is one of the major problems which in recent years has faced the medical fraternity. Many doctors, as well as naturopaths, claim that the foundations of overweight are laid in infancy. A common sight is the 'bonny' or overweight child snuffly with catarrh, suffering from recurrent colds and coughs, sore throats, adenoids, bronchial infections and stomach upsets. This state is almost entirely due to the excessively high intake of sweetened cereals, sweets, biscuits, iced lollies, chocolates and sweetened milky drinks which appear to be the major part of a child's diet – with an associated lack of fresh raw fruits, salads and vegetables.

Prevention of colds and influenza in children must consist of a radical change from this type of diet, a reduction of carbohydrate (sugar and starch) foods, and an introduction of pure fruit juices, fresh fruit, salads and vegetables. The difficulties of the child's dislike of salads etc. can gradually be overcome by a combination of patience, ingenuity and discipline.

The first necessity is to avoid eating between meals, and so encourage a natural healthy appetite at mealtimes; one which has not been masked by sweets or biscuits. A second necessity is to replace a milky bedtime drink with diluted fruit or vegetable juice. In practice, this one change in diet alone has often been found to make the difference between a bad night with no appetite for breakfast, and having a clear night with a good healthy hunger on waking.

Dr Bircher-Benner, the great Swiss nutritionist, came to the conclusion after extensive scientific research into nutrition, that a healthy person should take 50 per cent of his food raw, i.e. fresh raw vegetables, salads and fruits, and some raw whole-grain cereals. He wrote in great detail of his findings in research into diet, and laid down the principles of diet for children as well as for adults. He claimed:

'Three conditions determine the constitution, health and later lives of our children: heredity, mental and emotional experience in childhood, and diet.'

The Elderly

Another age-group which deserves special consideration is that of the elderly. Prohibited by reduced income, and perhaps by apathy, from preparing adequate meals, and with a slowing circulation, the retired person is susceptible to chills in cold or changeable weather. The state of health in the later period of life has its basis in the preceding years, when wise living may stave off normal physical degeneration for as long as possible.

However, commonsense measures must be mentioned. These include the maintenance of equable temperatures – avoiding drastic changes of temperature from one room to another – wearing of several thin layers of clothing of natural fibres instead of one thick layer, and by having as varied a diet as is feasible; not resorting, as – alas – so many elderly people do, to bread for breakfast, lunch and tea. If the elderly person has difficulty in chewing raw foods, these may be taken in the form of juice. If there is a poor appetite a herbal tea (see Agrimony in the section on remedies) may be advisable.

Vitamin Therapy

With regard to vitamins for the elderly, a multivitamin tablet is probably the most suitable. Recent research has shown that in a test group well over 50 per cent of elderly patients improved after only ten days of multivitamin therapy, and others after a longer period, and that the benefit was mainly lost about six weeks after the experiment was stopped.

The elderly person should keep as active as possible, both physically and mentally. A daily walk in the fresh air is advisable in good dry weather. A wise preventative medicine for the elderly is garlic, taken in capsule form. This not only builds up resistance to infection and helps to clear catarrh, but tends to reduce the cholesterol in the blood stream and, in some types of hypertension, can help lower blood-pressure. Of special benefit to the elderly is garlic's regulating effect on intestinal bacteria, by which it has been found to have beneficial action on many disorders of the digestive tract.

Herbal Teas
Herbal tisanes are often very helpful to the elderly, and can be quite acceptable to the palate. These herbal teas may become more than an habitual beverage, being taken for their specific action. For example, rose-hip tea is refreshing as well as being a source of vitamin C, and it will also stimulate the appetite. Lime-flower tea is a pleasant aid to lowering blood-pressure; Meadowsweet, alone or with Yarrow, will reduce acidity and help relieve stiff joints. Chamomile tea taken warm is sedative and soothing; taken cold, with a pinch of ginger, it relieves indigestion, colic and heartburn, and if required to stimulate the appetite should be taken cold an hour before a meal. Peppermint tea helps relieve indigestion.

Herbal teas may be obtained from health food stores, either in sachets, which may be infused as one does ordinary tea, or as herbs, in which case the normal method of infusion is one or two teaspoonsful to a teacupful of boiling water, covered and allowed to stand for five minutes. It may be sweetened with a little honey, which itself is a wholesome food, having healing, soothing and antiseptic qualities, and containing valuable trace elements such as iron, calcium, phosphate and manganese.

Thus it will be realized that there are a number of simple yet effective procedures which can easily become a part of daily life, and which will not only help to build up the body's natural resistance to disease, but will lay the foundations for general good health and wellbeing from childhood onwards.

2.

REMEDIAL TREATMENT

Whatever care may be taken with dietetic and other preventative measures, a cold or influenza may still develop. In such a case the herbal practitioner will advise rest in bed, in a warm but well-ventilated bedroom, with frequent hot herbal teas such as Elderflowers, Yarrow, and so on, to promote perspiration and to reduce the temperature.

A sponge down with cool or cold water will aid evaporation on the skin and thus assist in lowering temperature, or cold packs may be applied to chest, waist or throat, as specifically required. These are applied locally to reduce inflammation and congestion, and consist of cotton cloth of several thicknesses wrung out in cold water and applied firmly to the area, then covered with overlapping woollen material, which is fastened firmly in place.

After the initial coldness, which only lasts a moment or two, the pack should begin to warm. It may be replaced after half an hour by a fresh cold application, and this is repeated as necessary. The packs should not be used where there is considerable weakness or debility, and must be removed if they do not warm quickly. Rub the area briskly with a rough towel.

Fasting on fruit juices, especially lemon, grapefruit and orange, diluted with hot water and sweetened with a little honey, is advisable to aid the eliminative process.

Treatment of these infections varies with the differing stages, specific herbs being taken as indicated by symptoms. Prompt action at the first sign of a cold will often clear it completely overnight.

Warm Herbal Teas

This first stage of chill, in both colds and influenza, requires hot infusions of stimulating diaphoretics, perhaps with the addition of a little Cayenne when there is a deep penetrating chill; after perspiration has subsided and the temperature returned to normal, warm herbal teas such as Clivers or Boneset may be continued three or four times daily.

At this stage of influenza a persistent

cough, bronchial conditions or digestive disturbances may become evident, and herbs to deal with these are necessary. (See *Therapeutic Index*.) It is still wise to rest and to avoid fresh chills.

Continue with fruit juices, but if the appetite has returned fresh fruit may be eaten, and a gradual return to normal diet commenced with a home-made vegetable soup. Follow this with a good salad, then introduce a wider range of wholesome foods. During the restorative phase of an infection the body does not benefit from being overloaded with food, but requires a diet which is easy to digest and one containing vitamins and minerals. These assist the body in its recuperative action.

Convalescent Phase

The third stage of treatment can be regarded as the convalescent phase, with restitution of normal function and energy. The appetite may be returning, or may need the stimulus of herbal teas such as Sweet Flag, Gentian, or Tansy. Lethargy, inanition and depression, which so often follow influenza, may be felt now, and for these conditions there can be no finer remedies than Balm, Vervain, and Oats. A wineglassful of the indicated herbal tea, taken cool, will soon 'chase away melancholy', with perhaps an infusion of Rosemary at bedtime for restlessness and insomnia.

Catarrh or bronchial irritation may persist, for which there are many remedies, not only those mentioned in this book, but those described in detail in *Herbs to Ease Bronchitis* in this series.

Elimination
Throughout the illness, whether it be the brief duration of a cold or the longer term of influenza, elimination via the skin, kidneys or bowels is essential. Diaphoretic herbs assist skin action, while Clivers and Boneset also promote kidney activity; but it may be necessary to take either a herbal aperient or to have an enema to aid daily evacuation from the bowels.

The principles and purpose of herbal and naturopathic forms of treatment are directed towards aiding the natural healing force within the body, helping to build a stronger natural resistance to infection and to improving general health and vitality.

Although colds may occur even after a healthful regime has been followed for some time, their frequency, intensity and duration will be considerably reduced and the tiresome catarrh which so frequently follows colds will disappear.

Even if an attack of influenza is sustained it will be less devastating if the measures outlined in this book are followed vigorously, being shorter and with aftermath of depression or heart involvement either brief or absent. There can be no more successful and natural way of life than helping the body by providing it with correct nutritional and medicinal aid by taking simple natural remedies, and the reward will be improved health and vitality, and an ever-increasing *joie de vivre*.

AGRIMONY
(Agrimonia eupatoria)

The name of this common plant – which is found on waste ground and in hedgerows in Britain, Europe and North America – is of Greek origin, from *Argemone*, meaning 'a plant healing to the eyes', and its specific name from Mithridates Eupator, a king who gained a good reputation from his knowledge and use of herbs.

Growing up to 2ft (60cm) in height, Agrimony is a slender plant bearing small yellow flowers in tapering spikes, with deeply cut pinnate leaves. It is aromatic when bruised or crushed, the scent being described as similar to that of apricots. Indeed, it belongs to a sub-order of the *Rosaceae*, an Order which includes apricots, plums, cherries, apples, pears and many other fruits.

A mild astringent, diuretic and tonic, Agrimony has been known and used for centuries. Pliny described it as 'a herb of princely authority'; Dioscorides and Gerard

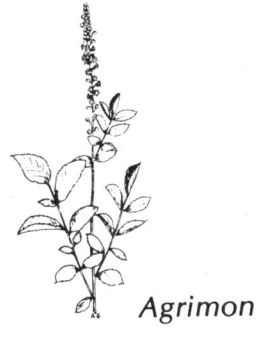

Agrimony

among many great physicians valued it highly. It has a wide range of uses, exerting its astringent effect on mucous membrane throughout the body. Taken in hot infusion, it has a diaphoretic effect, promoting good perspiration, and it is one of the plants which was used by North American Indians for fevers.

As a cold herbal tea, it becomes diuretic, increasing the flow of urine. The astringent properties render it valuable in acute or chronic diarrhoea, in dysentery, in cystitis, in chronic catarrh, and as a gargle for relaxed throat. It is beneficial in laryngitis and pharyngitis, and is one of the finest herbs for debility and lack of appetite, promoting the assimilation of food.

This remedy can be useful through all the stages of colds or influenza, where astringency is required, but it will not be beneficial if there is constipation or dryness of the throat, or a hard dry cough. Initially, it may be taken in hot infusion, a wineglassful every hour to bring about a good perspiration. A wineglassful of the cold infusion may be taken every two hours, or less often as required, for diarrhoea, and three times daily to have an effect on the kidneys.

For a loose, troublesome cough the cool infusion taken several times daily, with a final dose at bedtime, is recommended. Combined with sage in equal parts, it makes an excellent gargle.

Agrimony is considered by many herbalists to be incomparable during the convalescent stages of influenza or colds, when the appetite is negligible. It may be taken alone, a wineglassful one hour before a meal, or as in the following recipe.

Take 1oz. (25g) each of Agrimony, Gentian Root, Calumba Root and Centaury. Mix well, and make an infusion of 1oz. (25g) to 1pt. ($\frac{1}{2}$l) of boiling water. When cool, strain off the liquid and take a wineglassful one hour before each meal.

A good tonic is $\frac{1}{2}$oz. (10g) each of Agrimony, Balmony Herb, Gentian Root, Poplar Bark. Simmer gently for fifteen minutes in 3pt. ($1\frac{1}{2}$l) of water, keeping the pan closely covered. Allow to cool, and take a wineglassful three times daily. Agrimony may also be combined, in equal parts, with Dandelion Root as a tonic with influence on the liver. Do not sweeten tonic herbal teas.

4.

AVENS
(Geum urbanum)

Another member of the *Rosaceae*, Avens grows fairly commonly in hedgerows in Britain. It is an erect, slender plant growing up to 2ft (60cm) in height, its branched stems bearing a bright yellow flower. Its name comes from the Greek *geno*, 'to yield an agreeable fragrance', and it is claimed that an odour of cloves arises from the root when the plant is taken from the ground. The odour no doubt derives from the volatile oil present in all parts of the plant.

Avens is used by the modern herbal practitioner as a febrifuge and astringent. It is particularly indicated in diarrhoea and in

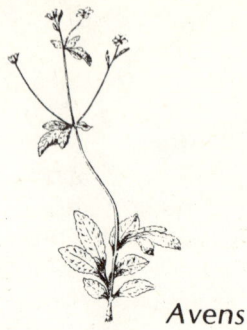

Avens

both ulcerative and catarrhal colitis, in which it is often combined with Agrimony. Avens has also been found useful in intermittent fevers, and thus is recommended as a hot infusion in the early stages of influenza, especially where there is loose catarrh and some diarrhoea.

It may be given in wineglassful doses every two or three hours. As the feverishness subsides, the infusion should be continued as a cool or cold tea three times daily right through the convalescent stages.

Persistent use of this herb will have a beneficial effect on the debility and lack of appetite which are common *sequelae* of influenza. As does Agrimony, this remedy helps promote appetite and assimilation of food.

The normal method of infusion for Avens is ½oz. (10g) of the powdered root to 1pt. (½l) of boiling water. Cover, allow to cool and strain off the liquid. Take hot or cold as indicated above.

5.

BALM
(Melissa officinale)

Known as Lemon Balm, this perennial is an easy plant to grow, and its young lemon-scented leaves in spring make a delicious tea. It is a Mediterranean plant from southern Europe, which has become naturalized in Britain. Its name is from the Greek *melissa*, meaning bee plant. The small white flowers prove a great attraction to bees, and formerly, according to Gerard, the leaves were rubbed on hives to keep the bees together and to attract others.

The healing properties of Balm have been known through the centuries; it was used by the Greeks as a soothing tea for fevers and for nerves. John Evelyn, the diarist, said: 'Balm is sovereign for the brain, strengthening the memory and powerfully chasing away melancholy.'

There is an Arabian proverb to the effect that Lemon Balm tea 'makes the heart merry and joyful'. It is diaphoretic, carminative and

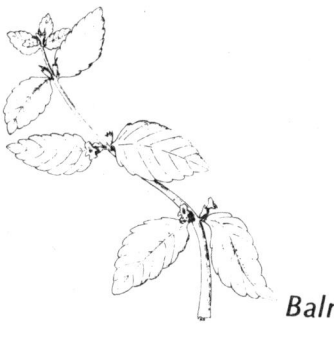

Balm

sedative, providing a cooling tea in both colds and influenza where there is a temperature, promoting perspiration and soothing both digestive system and nerves. For these conditions it should be taken in hot infusion, 1oz. (25g) of fresh leaves or ½oz. (10g) of dried leaves to 1pt. (½l) of boiling water.

Allow to infuse for fifteen minutes, keeping the vessel closely covered, and give a wineglassful every hour until a good perspiration occurs. Lemon Balm tea will ease griping pains in the bowels. It is a superb remedy during convalescence, soothing the nerves and digestion. Recent research has shown it to be beneficial in dyspepsia associated with nervous disorders and anxiety. In nervous disorders, especially with nightmares, it may be combined with Chamomile flowers, in equal parts.

Lemon Balm tea is a remedy *par excellence* for the post-influenza depression. A cold infusion may be taken several times daily, with a final dose just before retiring at night.

6.

BAYBERRY
(Myrica cerifera)

A North American shrub or small tree, Bayberry is the source of one of the main constituents of Composition Powder, and is a mild diaphoretic and astringent, with a tonic effect on the liver. It has a stimulating action on the circulation, and is given in infusion either alone or, preferably, with the addition

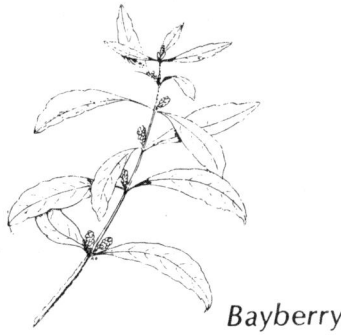
Bayberry

of a little Zingiber (ginger) in the first stage of colds, chills and acute fevers.

The infusion is made by pouring 1pt. ($\frac{1}{2}$l) of boiling water onto 1oz. (25g) of the powdered bark, and a small wineglassful should be taken every two or three hours until perspiration occurs, after which the frequency should be reduced. Large doses taken too often may cause a feeling of nausea.

The same infusion can be used as a gargle for either an acute or chronic sore throat. Its astringent properties also render this herb valuable in diarrhoea. It is a remedy which the herbalist uses for mucous colitis. Bayberry can be very effective in colds or influenza where the bronchial passages are involved, and where there is chilliness. Combine it in equal parts with Zingiber and Pleurisy Root (powdered), infuse $\frac{1}{2}$ teaspoonful in a teacupful of boiling water, with a pinch of Cayenne. This herb is, of course, available in the form of Composition Essence.

BONESET
(Eupatorium perfoliatum)

This plant is a native of North America, and was known to the Indians as ague-weed for its effectiveness in fevers. The name Boneset refers to its successful use in an American influenza which was called Breakbone fever because of the intense aching of the limbs during the fever. The flowering tops and leaves are used. Given in hot infusion, as hot as can be taken comfortably, as frequently as half-hourly, it will promote a profuse perspiration, lower the temperature and clear the cold quickly.

The specific indication for this remedy is influenza or fever with much aching in the limbs and soreness of muscles, and an intermittent fever with alternate feelings of heat and chilliness.

When the temperature is normal the herb may be given in warm or cool infusion, and will then act on stomach, liver and bowels, preventing gastric disturbance. It will also

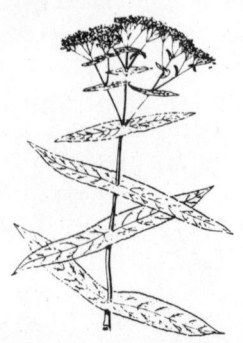

Boneset

soothe the nervous patient. It is effective when there is a loose cough and the chest is sore. As a cold infusion it is found to have tonic effect and can thus be continued into the convalescent stage of influenza. It is useful in catarrh, and also in mild attacks of muscular rheumatism.

The normal infusion of 1oz. (25g) to 1pt. ($\frac{1}{2}$l) of boiling water should be prepared, and a small wineglassful given each half-hour until perspiration has been promoted, then less frequently. Large doses continued frequently may have a purgative and emetic effect. When the patient is thoroughly chilled a hot infusion of $\frac{1}{2}$oz. (10g) each Boneset, Elder flowers and Yarrow, with a pinch of Cayenne powder or powdered Ginger, will speedily promote warmth and perspiration.

8.

CATMINT
(Nepeta cataria)

Catmint or catnep is a wild English plant, belonging to the *Labiatae* family. This is a family of about 2,500 species, found all over Europe in temperate climates and typified by square stems, two leaves opposite each other and lipped flowers. Not one of the whole natural order possesses any injurious properties; many are perfumed or aromatic: the Mints, Lavender, Patchouli, Basil, Thyme, Marjoram, medicinal plants such as Balm, Pennyroyal, Rosemary, Sage, Nettle, Peppermint.

Catmint is often found in gardens, and is

HERBS FOR COLDS AND 'FLU

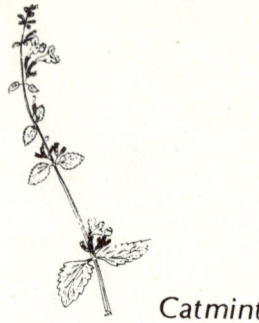

Catmint

beloved by cats, who will roll on and destroy any part of the plant which may be bruised. Yet there is an old couplet:

> If you set it, the cats will eat it,
> If you sow it, the cats don't know it,

the truth of which experience seems to confirm.

The flowering tops are used, and a hot infusion will promote a gentle free perspiration without increasing body heat. Taken at bedtime a good calm sleep will follow. Catmint has been found helpful in nervous headache, nervousness, and colic, and is beneficial in influenza for the patient who is restless.

NEVER boil this herb, as you will lose much of its value. Infuse it for ten minutes, keeping it closely covered. Small doses are advisable, as large doses given frequently may cause nausea and may have an emetic effect. One tablespoonful every two or three hours, and two teaspoonful for children will be adequate. Taken warm it will relieve the pain of colic, indigestion and menstruation. If sweetened with honey it will help to relieve coughs.

This herb was used as tea before that which we now use as a beverage was known to the western world and imported from China.

9.

CAYENNE
(Capsicum minimum)

This plant is from Africa, South America and tropical America. Its name is from the Greek *kapto*, meaning 'I bite'.

A fine stimulant, a small quantity added to herbal teas will reinforce their effect of equalizing the circulation. It acts beneficially upon the heart and extends its influence to the capillaries. It was used for centuries by the American Indians and Mexicans for all kinds of fevers.

This invaluable remedy is employed by herbalists in many compounds for chills, rheumatism, bronchial conditions, dyspepsia and flatulence, colic, and a wide range of complaints, and applied externally as a lotion

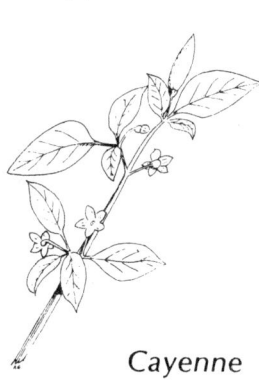

Cayenne

for lumbago and unbroken chilblains. Old herbalists used it locally for habitual cold feet.

Cayenne may be used in small doses with nerve agents such as Valerian, Verbena and Avena (Oats) for nervous depression, particularly the depression following influenza. Normally available in powdered form, the dose is 1 grain to a teacupful of boiling water, or of herbal infusion, or an infusion of 10 grains to a pint of boiling water. If the tincture is available the dose is 1 to 5 drops in hot water.

Cayenne may be used most effectively in the early stages of chills, especially where there is a feeling of chilliness in the back. It is also useful added to tonic medicines for debility, especially when the digestive system is affected.

10.

CLIVERS
(Galium aparine)

This common English plant belongs to the *Rubiaceae*, Madder family, one of the largest of natural orders comprising more than 2,800 species, some of which are of great value to man as food and medicine. It includes Cinchona (Peruvian Bark) in South America, Ipecacuanha and forty varieties of coffee (Brazil), the Indian plant Rubia Tinctoria (from which is prepared the red dye Madder), gardenias and many fragrant and beautiful flowers.

British species are all herbaceous plants; Ladies Bedstraw (*Galium vernum*) was used as

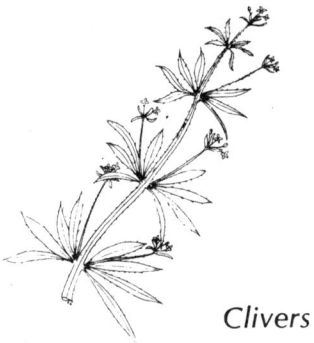

Clivers

a rennet to curdle milk and the seeds of Clivers roasted and used as coffee. Clivers grows abundantly in hedgerows in Britain; its long weak angular stalks with rosettes of narrow lancelike leaves are covered with tiny hooked bristles which enable it to cling to all other vegetation within reach. The name *aparine* comes from the Greek word *aparo*, meaning 'to seize'.

The remedy is particularly helpful as a hot infusion for colds in the head. It is a valuable diuretic, and is used by the herbal practitioner for a wide range of urinary conditions, including suppressed or scalding urine, when it may be combined with Marshmallow, Broom and other agents according to specific needs. For cystitis it is effective when combined with Marshmallow leaves or root. It has also been found valuable in skin conditions, and it has a gentle action on the bowels.

The normal infusion (1oz. (25g), 1 pt. ($\frac{1}{2}$l) boiling water) is taken hot in the early stages of a cold or influenza, especially when urine is scanty, and can be continued in warm infusion in wineglassful doses to act on kidneys and bowels. A warm infusion at bedtime can help to induce restful sleep when there is tendency to insomnia.

11.

COLTSFOOT
(Tussilago farfara)

This plant belongs to the natural order *Compositae*, an extensive family of about 10,000 species throughout the world, possessing both nutritional and medicinal properties. The family includes Lettuce, Chicory, Artichoke, Dandelion, Burdock, Wormwood, Southernwood, Tarragon, Dahlia, Sunflower, Chamomile, Marigold and many other familiar plants.

Coltsfoot is a common plant, indigenous to the temperate regions in Europe and Asia, its old name *Filius ante patrem* (son before the father) referring to the appearance of its bright yellow flowers which die down before the leaves are manifest. The herb grows on waste ground and on railway embankments, and is easily recognized as being the first wild

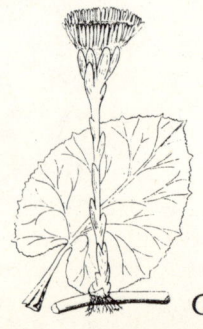

Coltsfoot

flower to appear in spring. The leaves are borne on long stalks, and are hoof-shaped with white felted hairs on the under-surface, and these are the part of the plant used in medicine.

This plant is one of the finest expectorants and demulcents available, and may be used specifically for spasmodic bronchial coughs. It is indicated for colds and influenza where a cough is present and when the sufferer has a history of bronchial conditions. A decoction is made by simmering 1oz. (25g) of the leaves in 1qt. (1l) of water down to 1pt. ($\frac{1}{2}$l). Take a wineglassful hot three times daily, or more often if the cough is troublesome.

This remedy may be combined with 1oz. (25g) of liquorice stick, decoction made as above, with a little honey or a slice of lemon added, and can be taken warm or cool. For an irritating cough combine this with White Horehound. (See *Therapeutic Index*.) Make a decoction, using $\frac{1}{2}$oz. (10g) of each, and add a little block juice (expressed liquorice root) or honey to sweeten. It may be given in spoonful doses frequently to children to relieve a spasmodic cough.

The Latin name *Tussilago* means 'Cough dispeller' and coltsfoot has well been described as 'nature's best herb for the lungs'.

12.

ECHINACEA
(Echinacea angustifolia)

Growing to about 2ft (60cm) in height,

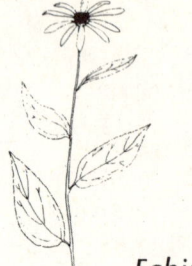

Echinacea

Echinacea – also known as Black Sampson – is a native of America and belongs to the *Compositae* family. It is a mild diaphoretic and is antiseptic.

This remedy has long been used both internally and externally for its antiseptic properties, and is considered by modern herbalists to be a fine antibiotic. Valuable in fevers and septic conditions, and for abscesses, boils and carbuncles, it is also used successfuly in tonsillitis and pharyngitis, and has been of great service in naso-pharyngeal catarrh. Echinacea has also been found to improve digestion and appetite.

It may be taken in hot infusion to promote perspiration and to improve peripheral circulation, and is advisably continued as a cool infusion for the duration of the illness in influenza, or where there is any tendency to septic infections.

The infusion is made by pouring a teacupful of boiling water onto a teaspoonful of powdered root and allowing it to stand (covered) for half an hour. Strain off the liquid and take 1 tablespoonful up to six times daily in the early stages, and subsequently three times daily as a regular dose.

The dose of the tincture is five to ten drops in a little water. This remedy is more specific for influenza than for the common cold.

13.

ELDER
(Sambucus nigra)

Belonging to *Caprifoliaceae*, Woodbine family, a natural order which mostly grows in the northern hemisphere extending from California to China and including Honeysuckle and species known for their beautiful flowers, this small tree is native to Britain and grows abundantly in hedges and old gardens. The name Elder comes from the Anglo-Saxon word *aeld* meaning 'fire'; an allusion to the habit of using the hollow young stems to blow up a fire. This tree was known to the Greeks, to Pliny, and was reputed to be a favourite remedy of the great Hippocrates.

John Evelyn, the diarist, said:

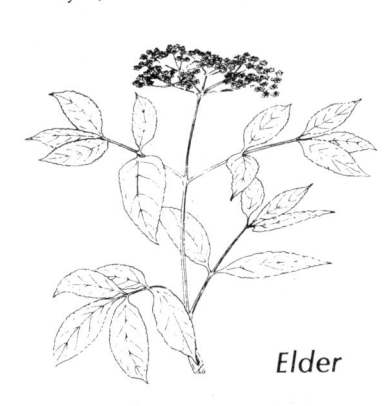

Elder

If the medicinal properties of the leaves, bark, and berries were thoroughly known I cannot tell what our countryman could ail for which he could not find a remedy from every hedge, either for sickness or wounds.

The flowers are used for colds and influenza, and may be used alone or even more effectively combined with Peppermint herb: 1oz. (25g) to 1pt. ($\frac{1}{2}$l) of boiling water, or 1oz. (25g) Elder flowers, 1oz. (25g) Peppermint herb and $\frac{1}{2}$oz. (10g) Yarrow herb, to 1qt. (1l) boiling water. Drink a wineglassful frequently. Be sure to keep the infusion closely covered, to avoid loss of valuable volatile oils and other constituents in the steam.

For influenza, take $\frac{1}{2}$oz. (10g) Elder flowers and $\frac{1}{2}$oz. (10g) Peppermint; infuse for half an hour in a warm place in 1pt. ($\frac{1}{2}$l) of boiling water. Strain off the liquid, sweeten with a little honey and drink half the quantity as hot as possible on going to bed. This will induce free perspiration (hence the need to drink it in bed) and so help to clear the influenza quickly. The remainder may be taken hot a few hours later if required.

When combined with Peppermint this remedy is found helpful for colic and flatulence, and when taken with herbs such as Hyssop it has a beneficial effect on the lungs, clearing mucus and soothing irritation.

Elder flowers have long been used as a cool lotion in skin conditions, eruptive diseases such as measles (use $\frac{1}{2}$oz. (10g) to 1 pt. ($\frac{1}{2}$l) boiling water, cool and bathe with the strained liquid), and may be used in the bath in cases of irritability of skin and nerves. A weak lotion may be used to bathe the eyes.

Elderberry wine has long been accounted a good remedy for coughs and colds, taken in hot water, as also has Elderberry syrup and Elderberry rob. The rob is made with fresh ripe berries, picked from the stalks. Stew very gently with one-fifth their weight in sugar until the liquid has evaporated to the thickness of honey. Strain this, allow to cool, and bottle. This is soothing to the chest and will promote perspiration if half a tablespoonful is taken in a glassful of hot water at bedtime.

To make Elderberry syrup, stew fresh berries gently in a little water until the juice flows. Strain, add a few cloves and whole ginger – $\frac{1}{2}$oz. (10g) to 1 gal. (4.5l) – then boil gently for one hour. Strain and bottle when cool. Take a small wineglassful in hot water, with a little honey.

14.

GARLIC
(Allium sativum)

This valuable plant has been known since earliest recorded times, and together with onion and leek was cultivated in ancient Egypt for food. It was praised for its medicinal properties by many ancient writers such as Galen and Pliny, and by the English herbalist, Turner, *circa* 1548.

Garlic is a superb antiseptic; its value cannot be over-emphasized. The plant contains a volatile oil rich in sulphur (which provides the pungent odour), a mucilage and other constituents. It is diaphoretic,

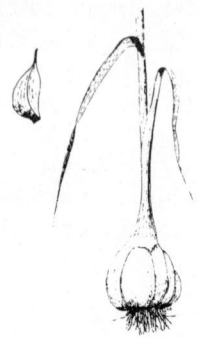

Garlic

expectorant, antiviral and antiseptic. It acts on all mucous membranes, the lining of mouth, throat, nasal and respiratory passages, and the alimentary system.

Garlic is specifically beneficial for chronic bronchitis, but is invaluable for recurrent colds, catarrh, coughs, asthma and other bronchial conditions. It gives protection against infection; therefore it should be used continuously in a preventative role rather than taken temporarily during an acute infection.

The fresh bulb is the part used, and it can be made into syrup by slicing, covering with boiling water, allowing to stand for twelve hours, then adding sugar to make it to the consistency of syrup. A little vinegar in which Caraway and Fennel seeds have been boiled will remove the odour if added to the syrup. This may be taken in spoonful doses to ease a cough and promote expectoration, and for other lung disorders.

The easiest method of using Garlic medicinally is to take the Garlic oil capsules, which are deodorized. One before each meal or three at bedtime, taken regularly during winter, will most certainly help to reduce infection. Garlic may also be used in food, when the odour can be removed from the breath by chewing Parsley, Mint, Basil or Thyme.

Recent research has shown that garlic has the power of reducing the cholesterol level in the blood, and of lowering high blood-pressure.

15.

GOLDEN ROD
(Solidago virgaurea)

This is the only British species, a common plant up to 30in. (75cm) tall, bearing terminal clusters of bright yellow flowers on roughish angular stems. Its names is from the Latin *solidare*, meaning to 'make whole', an allusion to its old uses in healing wounds.

The therapeutic actions are diaphoretic, antiseptic, diuretic and carminative. The leaves and flowers are used. A hot infusion is valuable and quick in promoting perspiration in influenza, and is good when there is

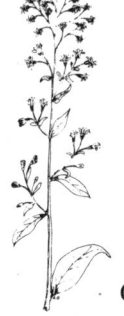

Golden Rod

chilliness alternating with heat, bouts of sneezing and irritable nose.

Its antiseptic qualities render this herb valuable for all sluggish or septic conditions of the upper respiratory tract, and specifically useful for catarrhal conditions. It contains astringent properties, which will act on mucous membranes and may thus be used both as a medicine and as a local spray or gargle for catarrh of nose and throat and for laryngitis. It has been used successfully in cystitis, as a cool infusion. It is a good remedy for most digestive disturbances, especially flatulent dyspepsia.

The normal infusion of 1oz. (25g) to 1pt. ($\frac{1}{2}$l) should be taken in wineglassful doses three times daily or more often in acute conditions.

16.

WHITE HOREHOUND
(Marrubium vulgare)

This indigenous plant, which grows on waste ground and by roadsides, is common all over Europe. It was valued by the Egyptians and the Romans, and was recommended by Gerard. In England it was cultivated in cottage gardens, and used for making cough candy and herbal tea.

In addition to its well-known efficacy in coughs and bronchial conditions, White Horehound is most effective in hot infusion for colds, promoting a free perspiration and to some extent stimulating the flow of urine.

Make the normal infusion of 1oz. (25g) to 1pt. ($\frac{1}{2}$l), allow to stand for at least ten minutes

White Horehound

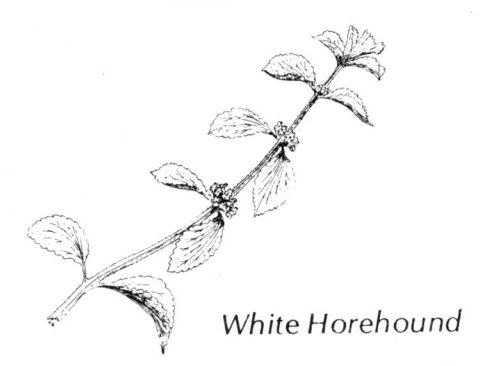

and take a wineglassful hot every two or three hours.

This remedy is indicated in colds associated with bronchial conditions, particularly chronic states where there may be a non-productive cough. It has also been of great service in whooping cough, combined with Ginger, and is excellent for children's coughs. A smaller dose is then advisable, according to age.

17.

HYSSOP
(Hyssopus officinalis)

A member of the *Labiatae*, this plant grows extensively in Southern Europe, but is not native to Britain. It was known to the Greeks, from which its name *azob* arose, meaning 'holy herb'. It is referred to in the Scriptures: 'Purge me with Hyssop and I shall be clean.' It grows wild in Mediterranean regions, and is cultivated in Germany, France, India and the U.S.S.R. Hyssop is an attractive, aromatic plant, ground up to 2ft (60cm) tall, with spikes

Hyssop

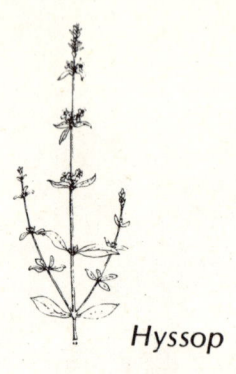

of blue flowers and narrow leaves.

The whole plant contains a volatile oil, and is diaphoretic, expectorant and sedative in its action. It is specifically valuable in colds and bronchitis, and is most effective in chronic nasal catarrh. Used alone in hot infusion for colds, it is often combined with Horehound to relieve coughs and for bronchial catarrh (taken as either hot or warm infusion), when it will work to expel mucus. A cool infusion is often used as a gargle, when a few sage leaves may be added to the herb on infusing.

The sedative action of Hyssop renders it a valuable herb to use for patients suffering from anxiety. The leaves may be applied to bruises, to reduce the inflammation and pain.

18.

LIME FLOWERS
(Tilia platyphyllos)

These are found on a British tree, which grows in the north temperate zone. The flowers contain a volatile oil, which causes delightful

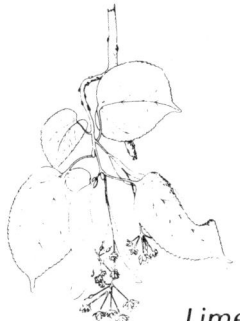

Lime Flowers

perfuming of the air when the tree is in flower.

The whole tree is most useful, its wood being ideal for carving; it never becomes worm-eaten. The inner bark yields fibres which have been used to make matting and baskets, the sap in spring affords sugar, and finally the leaves and shoots are mucilaginous and may be used in poultices.

The flowers are diaphoretic, diuretic, sedative and mildly astringent. They constitute one of the popular tisanes of France. Given as hot infusion this remedy is most successful in feverish colds when there is frequent sneezing. It may be combined for this purpose with Elder flowers.

As a cool infusion Lime is sedative, helpful in nervous or hysterical conditions. It has been found beneficial in migraine, taken in cool infusion during and after an attack, but it is wise to seek the advice of a qualified herbal practitioner to undertake more comprehensive treatment.

The quality for which Lime blossom tea is perhaps now more widely known is the beneficial effect on hypertension; raised blood-pressure. The tea should be taken in place of ordinary tea and coffee, as both a warm and a cool drink. Sweetened with a little honey this may be enjoyed as a pleasant beverage.

19.

MEADOWSWEET
(Filipendula ulmaria)

The plant belongs to *Rosaceae*, an extensive family of over 1,000 species, which includes the rose species, fruits such as Apple, Pear, Quince, Peach, Nectarine, Apricot, Raspberry, Blackberry, Almonds, and others; medicinal plants such as Agrimony, Avens and Hawthorn.

Meadowsweet, or Queen-of-the-meadow, is a common native British herb, growing profusely in hedgerows, by roadsides and in moist places. From June to September its delicate tufts of creamy-white flowers perfume the air. The whole plant is used in infusion, it is a stomachic, mild astringent, and mildly antiseptic.

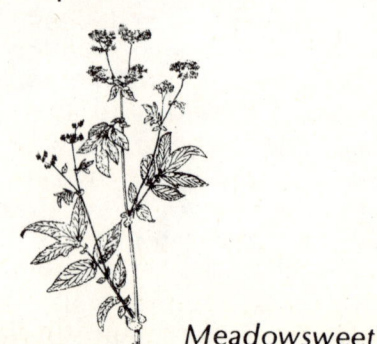

Meadowsweet

A hot infusion of the fresh tops will induce perspiration, and a warm infusion of the whole herb will relieve the discomfort of acute cystitis. The astringent properties cause this herb to be especially helpful in mild diarrhoea and dysentery, and in children's diarrhoea.

Meadowsweet is excellent for a wide range of digestive disturbances, particularly acidity, heartburn and dyspepsia, when it may be used in equal parts with Balm or with Marshmallow leaves. A cool infusion sweetened with honey is a good drink for invalids. A wineglassful is the usual dose, taken three times daily or more often in acute conditions. Smaller doses of about a tablespoonful may be given to children, depending on age.

20.

OATS
(Avena sativa)

There are many varieties of this cereal, ranging from *Avena siberica*, a native of Siberia to *A.filiformis*, indigenous to New Zealand. The nutritive qualities of oats have long been known, and the herbal physician has often recommended them as a nerve tonic during convalescence. At such time they may be taken as a gruel, and may also be used in cooking.

Oats are tonic to the nervous system, to blood, hair, nails and teeth, and were considered a remedy for rickets. The dehusked seed of the plant is the part used, and contains starch, protein, vitamins B and E, and the minerals potassium and phosphorus.

Medicinally oats are given in tincture and fluid extract, and prescribed specifically for melancholy and depressive states, when they may be combined with Scullcap or other nervines, and for general debility. They exert a mild tonic effect on heart muscle. *Avena* is considered by many to be the finest remedy for nervous exhaustion and debility following prostrating illnesses.

Oats influence the brain and nervous system, and help to induce sleep. The gruel is made by boiling 1oz. (25g) of oatmeal in 3pt. (1½l) of water until reduced to 1qt. (1l); strain off the liquid and add honey to sweeten, and a little lemon if desired, or add black treacle, or a few raisins.

A tea may be made by soaking a teaspoonful of oats in a cupful of hot water for at least ten minutes, then straining it and sweetening with a little honey. Take this at least once daily.

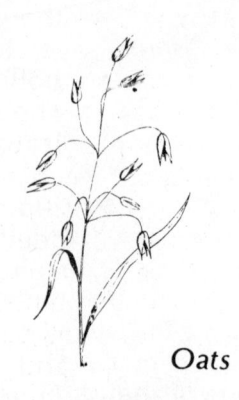

Oats

PLEURISY ROOT
(Asclepias tuberosa)

This plant is indigenous to North America, the name arising from its therapeutic value in pleurisy.

Pleurisy root is diaphoretic, expectorant, antispasmodic and carminative, directing its main influence towards the lungs. It reduces inflammation, expelling mucus and easing difficult breathing. This remedy is indicated in colds or influenza where there is a previous history of lung conditions such as pneumonia, or even more specifically where pain is felt in the region of the lungs on breathing.

The cut root is made into a decoction, prepared by adding ½oz. (10g) to 1pt. (½l) of water, bringing to the boil and simmering very gently until the volume is reduced to ¾pt. (400ml). A small wineglassful may be taken warm every three hours until relief is obtained. An infusion of the powdered root is made by adding one teaspoonful of powder to a teacup of boiling water, and allowing it to stand for one hour.

To promote perspiration, a small wineglassful of either decoction or infusion with a little Composition essence or powdered Ginger root added may be taken every hour until free perspiration has taken place. It may also be combined with Angelica and Sassafras root, in equal parts, to promote perspiration in fevers and pleurisy. It is excellent for children's fevers, given every

Pleurisy Root

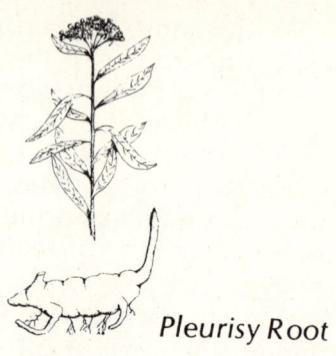

hour or two in small doses, according to age. If the child is restless, a little Scullcap should be added to the infusion.

Pleurisy root is quickly effective, and is advisably given in small doses as frequently as indicated above, with the dosage reduced gradually to three times daily when perspiration has taken place, pain has eased and the temperature is normal. It will then continue to assist expectoration. In pulmonary congestions add a pinch of Cayenne powder to each cupful.

22.

ROSEMARY
(Rosmarinus officinalis)

This evergreen shrub, with its narrow leaves and pale blue flowers, belongs to the *Labiatae*, a valuable family of medicinal and aromatic plants. It thrives on dry, rocky soil near to the sea in Mediterranean countries extending eastwards from Spain, and grows well in this country in a sheltered situation.

Rosemary has long been considered to be

ROSEMARY

one of the most powerful remedies to stimulate and strengthen the nervous system. Known to the ancient healers, it was reputed to improve the memory. Much symbolism was attached to it, mainly as an expression of fidelity; it adorned churches, and was used in religious ceremonies. Brides and wedding guests wore it and it was featured in wedding bouquets.

There is an old saying: 'Where rosemary flourishes the women rule.' The main goodness lies in the flowering tops, with secondary value in the leaves and stems. The whole plant contains a volatile oil, and care must be taken to avoid vapour escaping whilst infusing the herb. Rosemary tea, infused from the young tops (both flowers and leaves), when taken warm will induce gentle perspiration, and provides an excellent remedy for colds, colic, headaches, and nerves. It has a gentle tonic action on the heart.

In colds or influenza Rosemary should be taken in the early stages as a hot or warm infusion, and may be continued as a cooling tea when there is restlessness, nervousness

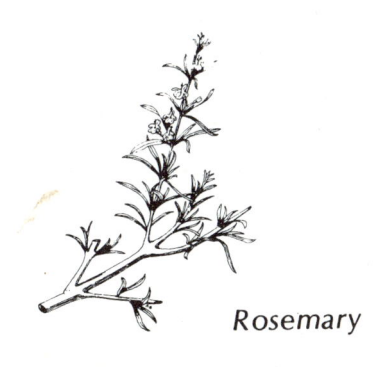

Rosemary

and insomnia. The combination of Rosemary with Sage and Vervain, in equal parts, makes a powerful antiseptic drink, which is invaluable in fevers.

This herb has a reputation for value in a wide range of conditions, including external application to wounds, bites and stings. Another external use is as a hair tonic, and the oil makes an excellent insecticide. It can be beneficial in high blood-pressure, taken as an infusion three times daily. The normal infusion is 1oz. (25g) to 1pt. ($\frac{1}{2}$l). Cover the vessel closely, and take 1 wineglassful frequently to promote perspiration, or as required for headaches or nervous conditions.

23.

SAGE
(Salvia officinalis)

The name comes from the Latin *salvere*, 'to be well', 'to save'. This extremely valuable plant grows in numerous varieties in Mediterranean countries, extending eastwards from Spain to Greece and beyond; growing also in China and Mexico.

Sage was well known to the Greeks and Romans, and widely used in the Middle Ages. There was one Latin proverb which asked: 'Why should a man die whilst sage grows in his garden?', and the great English herbalist Gerard said:

> Sage is singularly good for the head and brain, it quickeneth the senses and memory, strengthens the sinews, restoreth health to

those that have the palsy, and taketh away shakey trembling.

Common Sage, the variety used medicinally, also known as Red Sage, is grown in gardens in Britain as a culinary herb. The leaves are used, the volatile oil in the plant being the active principle.

Sage tea taken hot in small, frequent doses is effective for head colds, feverishness, delirium, biliousness, sore throat and quinsy, and is helpful in measles, joint pains and in nervous headaches. It has also been found good for digestive ailments, especially with flatulence. It long had a reputation of controlling excessive perspiration at night. The infusion may be used as a gargle in any form of sore throat.

This herb is specific in colds and influenza where there is a previous history of recurrent sore throats, and indeed its continued use to improve the throat conditions after the cold has cleared, would be well advised. In this instance a wineglassful of cool infusion taken two or three times daily, and also used as a gargle, will have long-term benefits.

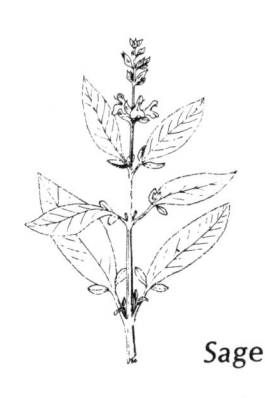

Sage

The infusion is made by adding 1 teaspoonful of leaves to ½pt. (¼l) boiling water, covering the vessel closely, or infuse ½oz. (10g) of the leaves with the juice of one lemon for half an hour in 1qt. (1l) of boiling water. Add honey to taste. The plain infusion may be inhaled for congestion in the nose and head.

24.

SWEET FLAG
(Acorus calamus)

An aquatic reed-like plant which grows by the edges of ditches, waterways, ponds and lakes. It is indigenous in most European countries and in Central Asia. Sweet Flag was known to Pliny and Dioscorides, and was first grown in England by Gerard in 1596.

This remedy is diaphoretic and carminative, and its specific use is for colic with flatulence. Its greatest benefit is exerted on the digestive system, aiding digestion, dissipating fermentation, relieving dyspepsia, reducing acidity and stimulating the appetite. It is one of the finest herbs for digestive disturbances during convalescence, and a nutritive tonic in debility and loss of appetite. It has also been found effective in ague and fevers, and for nervous complaints.

Sweet Flag is used as a decoction, as infusion of the powdered root, as fluid extract or tincture. For a decoction, add 1oz. (25g) of cut root to 1½pt. (¾l) water, bring to boil and simmer until reduced to 1pt. (½l). Doses of a wineglassful may be taken hot quite frequently to promote a gentle perspiration. An infusion is made by adding one teaspoonful of powder to a large teacupful of boiling water. Leave to stand for fifteen minutes, closely covered. A little powdered ginger may be added to the warm infusion, when this is required for flatulence or colic. Take in tablespoonful doses. It may be combined with Meadowsweet for acidity and dyspepsia.

A tonic to increase appetite can be made from 15 to 30 drops of tincture or fluid extract in a little water. This is also helpful for general debility. The infusion used as a gargle will ease a sore throat, and applied externally will relieve the inflammation of wounds and burns. It also has antibiotic properties, rendering it a good agent for influenza and other fevers.

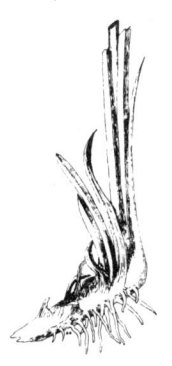

Sweet Flag

TANSY
(Tanacetum vulgare)

This is a very common plant, growing on waste ground. In August it produces flat corymbs or discs of bright yellow small flowers, and grows up to 3ft (90cm) in height. It is aromatic, with a camphor-like odour. The name Tansy is reputed to come from the Greek word *athanaton*, which means 'immortal'.

The herb has a long and interesting history. It was used to strew the floors of churches and castles, was grown in gardens for its brightness and its culinary values, was transformed into Tansy cakes and yellow dye. For centuries it has had a wide range of uses, being tonic and stimulant. It is well known for its influence in relieving tardy menstruation when this is due to cold or chill, mitigating much of the discomfort; but it is not effective in delays due to any other cause and should not be given when pregnancy is suspected.

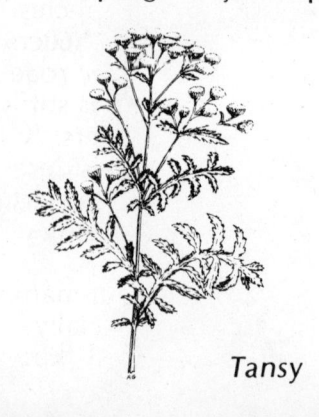

Tansy

A hot infusion is valuable in feverish colds and fevers, and is used in digestive disturbances, especially when associated with flatulence. Taken as a cool tea it is a general tonic for lassitude and debility, poor appetite and a tired feeling during convalescence. Tansy is soothing in nervous conditions.

The dose must always be small, a tablespoonful of the infusion being sufficient. This may be taken every three hours to promote perspiration, then at less frequent intervals. As a cool tonic the same-sized dose three times daily before meals will suffice. The infusion is made by adding a teaspoonful of the herb to 1pt. ($\frac{1}{2}$l) of boiling water and allowing it to stand, well-covered, for half an hour. This infusion may also be used externally as a fomentation to sprained or rheumatic joints, or in sciatica.

26.

VERVAIN
(Verbena officinalis)

This is the only British species, a common plant growing up to 2ft (60cm) high and found on waste ground, by roadsides and in pastures. This perennial has stiff stems which carry small pale lilac flowers. Known also as Herb of Grace, it was considered in ancient times to possess great healing virtues, and was regarded as a holy plant, being used to sweep the altars.

Once thought to benefit mankind in every illness, Vervain is especially valuable in influenza and fevers of all kinds, including

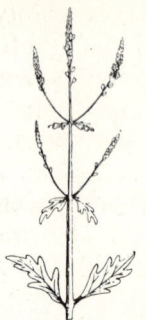

Vervain

remittent fever. Its specific indication is in the depression and debility following such diseases. Vervain is beneficial in nervous disorders, mental stress, and exerts some influence on the heart. It has been used successfully in liver conditions and biliary colic, and for chronic lung conditions.

Vervain is one of the many remedies used by the herbal practitioner in the treatment of hay fever. Take ½oz. (10g) each of Vervain, Sage, Yarrow and White Horehound, simmer gently for fifteen minutes in 1qt. (1l) of water. A wineglassful may be taken three or more times daily. Dietetic measures are necessary in this condition, and for obstinate cases the advice of a herbal practitioner should be sought.

The normal infusion may be prepared of 1oz. (25g) herb to 1pt. (½l) of boiling water, and taken hot three or four times daily, in wineglassful doses, to promote a gentle perspiration. The same infusion taken cold three times daily will be invaluable in all states of depression, melancholy and debility during convalescence.

Vervain may be combined with Scullcap

and Oats for nervous debility; take ½oz. (10g) of each and simmer gently for ten minutes in 1½pt. (¾l) of water. If one were limited in the selection of herbs with which to treat influenza, Vervain would be the first choice, as it is mildly diaphoretic, and thus can be used in the first stages. It is useful for the liver and is a wonderful remedy for mental exhaustion and post-influenzal depression.

27.

YARROW
(Achillea millefolium)

This is a fine remedy for the first stages of colds and fevers; take in hot infusion, either alone or combined with Elderflowers and Peppermint. It is a common wayside plant growing up to 18in. (45cm) high, with finely cut leaves and corymbs or discs of white or pink flowers from June to September. It is an aromatic plant. Used in ancient times externally to heal wounds, it is reputed to be named after Achilles, the Greek warrior.

Yarrow is diaphoretic, antipyretic, diuretic

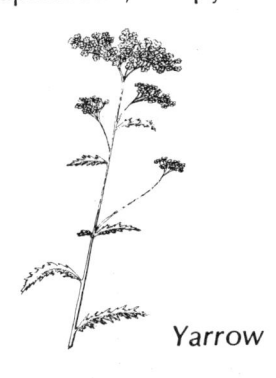

Yarrow

and astringent; it will be found valuable for producing a good perspiration and is good in many kidney disorders and in diarrhoea.

The infusion must be kept closely covered, and taken hot to promote perspiration; or cool three or four times daily for kidney conditions, diarrhoea and headaches. The infusion may be sweetened with a little honey. Add a teaspoonful of Composition essence or a pinch of Cayenne to a wineglassful of hot infusion when the patient feels chilled; or if the chest is affected add the expressed liquorice root known as block juice.

The cool infusion may be taken with Lime flowers in nervous disorders and raised blood-pressure.

THERAPEUTIC INDEX

Aching limbs, Boneset.
Acidity, Meadowsweet.
Antiseptic, Echinacea, Garlic, Golden Rod, Meadowsweet, Rosemary.
Anxiety, Hyssop.
Appetite, loss of, Agrimony, Avens, Echinacea, Sweet Flag, Tansy.
Asthma, Garlic.
Biliousness, Sage, Vervain.
Blood-pressure, Garlic, Lime Flowers, Rosemary, Yarrow.
Bowels, Balm, Boneset, Clivers.
Bronchial conditions, Bayberry, Coltsfoot, Elder, Garlic, Golden Rod, Horehound, Hyssop, Pleurisy Root, Vervain, Yarrow.
Bruises, Hyssop.
Catarrh, Agrimony, Avens, Boneset,

THERAPEUTIC INDEX 63

Echinacea, Garlic, Golden Rod, Hyssop.
Chills, Bayberry, Cayenne, Golden Rod.
Colds in head, Clivers, Sage.
Colic, Catmint, Cayenne, Elder, Rosemary, Sweet Flag, Vervain.
Colitis, Avens, Bayberry.
Convalescence, Avens, Balm, Meadowsweet, Oats, Sweet Flag, Tansy.
Cough, Agrimony, Boneset, Catmint, Coltsfoot, Elder, Garlic, Horehound, Hyssop.
Cough, spasmodic, Coltsfoot.
Cystitis, Agrimony, Clivers, Golden Rod, Meadowsweet.
Debility, Agrimony, Cayenne, Oats, Sweet Flag, Tansy, Vervain.
Depression, Balm, Cayenne, Oats, Vervain.
Diarrhoea, Agrimony, Avens, Meadowsweet, Yarrow.
Digestive disturbance, Balm, Boneset, Catmint, Cayenne, Golden Rod, Meadowsweet, Sage, Sweet Flag, Tansy.
Dysentery, Agrimony, Meadowsweet.
Dyspepsia, Balm, Cayenne, Golden Rod, Meadowsweet, Sweet Flag.
Flatulence, Cayenne, Elder, Golden Rod, Sage, Sweet Flag, Tansy.
Hay fever, Vervain.
Headache, Catmint, Rosemary, Sage, Yarrow.
Heart, Cayenne, Oats, Rosemary, Vervain.
Hysteria, Lime Flowers.
Infection, to protect against, Garlic.
Influenza, Agrimony, Avens, Bayberry, Balm, Boneset, Catmint, Cayenne, Clivers, Coltsfoot, Echinacea, Elder, Golden Rod, Pleurisy Root, Rosemary, Sage, Sweet Flag, Vervain.

Insomnia, Clivers, Oats, Rosemary.
Intermittent fever, Boneset, Vervain.
Kidneys, Agrimony, yarrow.
Laryngitis, Agrimony.
Liver, Agrimony, Bayberry, Boneset, Vervain.
Memory, Rosemary, Sage.
Migraine, Lime Flowers.
Nerves, Balm, Catmint, Elder, Lime Flowers, Oats, Rosemary, Sweet Flag, Vervain, Yarrow.
Nightmares, Balm.
Night perspiration, Sage.
Pain, Catmint, Pleurisy Root.
Pain, griping, Balm.
Restlessness, Catmint, Rosemary.
Rheumatism, muscular, Boneset.
Rheumatism of joints, Sage, Tansy.
Septic conditions, Echinacea.
Skin, Clivers, Elder.
Sneezing, Golden Rod, Lime Flowers.
Throat, Echinacea, Golden Rod, Sage, Sweet Flag.
Urinary disorders, Clivers, Horehound.
Whooping cough, Coltsfoot, Garlic, Horehound.